Keto Meal Plan – The Art of Keto Meal Plan

A Complete Beginner's Guide to Simple, Quick & Delicious Ketogenic Recipes in 10 Minutes or Less to Burn Fat and Loss Weight

By: Anthony Fung & Jason T. William

Disclaimer

No part of this publication may be reproduced or transmitted in any form or by any means, mechanical or electronic, including photocopying or recording, or by any information storage or retrieval system, or transmitted by email without permission in writing from the publisher.

While all attempts have been made to verify the information provided in this publication, neither the author nor the publisher assumes any responsibility for errors, omissions, or contrary interpretations of the subject matter herein.

This book is for entertainment purposes only. The views expressed are those of the author alone and should not be taken as expert instructions of commands. The reader is responsible for his or her own actions.

Adherence to all applicable laws and regulations, including international, federal, state and local governing professional licensing, business practices, advertising, and all other aspects of doing business in the US, Canada, or any other jurisdiction is the sole responsibility of the purchaser or reader.

Neither the author nor the publisher assumes any responsibility or liability whatsoever on the behalf of the purchaser or reader of these materials.

Any perceived slight of any individual or organization is purely unintentional.

Table of Contents

Bonus (Highly Recommended)

How do you compress decades in to days? It is by learning and modelling from people who have already walked the talk and done what you want to do.

If you want to lose weight, gain the body that you so deserve, achieve self-confidence and self-esteem that you never thought you had. I have a very special offer for you.

Visit this link:

http://bit.ly/leanbellyhack

watch a FREE video on a life changing transformation that could happen to you in 3 days, 1 month, 3 months and 1 year from now. You do not have to be the same today after watching this video, only so by choice.

http://bit.ly/leanbellyhack

Introduction

The keto meal? Where is that coming from again? You may wonder. Is it the latest junk food in the market today? No, I can assure you that you are far from the answer. Or is it a meal that makes you stronger? Now, you are getting warmer.

The keto meal is a strict diet that helps you burn fat a lot more efficiently. As you might have already known, fat can cause a lot of health issues, most especially when they clog in your blood streams. If you did not already know that, now you know. I give that to you as a free tip, no extra charge. Winks!

To make thing a lot more fun, the keto meal when undertaken properly can effect changes like weight loss, improved health, fight cancer, diabetes, and I could keep going with the list. And not also forgetting, it makes you stronger, not with muscles or anything out of the usual, but stronger in your health.

For you to be able to get the full benefits of the keto diet there are a couple of things you need to know. Most especially on what you are free to eat and the types of foods you need to run at 440 km/h away from. Just kidding, but seriously there are some foods you need to avoid.

Apart from what you can eat and all what not, the main idea of this book is to get you some really great keto recipes. And that is what I am going to do. But first as a beginner that you are, or not, I need to make sure that you are aware of the basics. So, without further ado, let us jump start into all what you need to know about keto diet and get you started with some really great recipes. Adieu!

Chapter 1: What is Keto Dieting?

What is the fuss about keto diet everyone seems to be talking about these days? Well, the fuss is all about the health benefits of a keto diet. Keto diet is simply a diet that is low in carbohydrates, but significantly high in proteins and fats. Keto diet is a short way of saying the full Ketogenic diet.

I know right! Just protein and fat, although that is no excuse to eat all the bacon in the world. Keto diet is great and has lots of health benefits, which we would be discussing later in the book. You may have heard about the keto diet from a friend, or you probably saw it on TV, the truth is keto diet would do better to you that you can possibly imagine.

Many times, we just eat food for our belly without even taking a second to imagine what our body really needs. Being obsessed or having fats at the wrong places may be as a result of the wrong food that we eat. Exercise helps a lot, but while exercising, combine it with the right dieting can go a long way.

Keto diet is a type of diet that pays attention to reducing excessive fat in your body. Did you know that when you eat, especially carbohydrate food, it is converted to glycogen which is stored under your skin? I guess by now you can now draw the dots that connect keto diet with low carbohydrate in the diet.

So, in essence, the Keto diet is a type of diet that can really help you burn those fats. It is healthy and will not require you cutting drastically low on your overall diet - starving yourself. Your meals can still be completely whole, but low in carbohydrates and you can still burn those fats and burn them really fast. It all depends on how badly you want it to happen.

Basically, there are lots of hype out there about the keto diet. Half of it might be true and might not be true; it all depends on what you have heard. But you can be sure that you have found the right book that states only facts and proven points. You can also rest your mind that everything you read in this book can be proven scientifically and not rumors or what people believe to be true.

Now, let's get a little into science a bit. You see, when you are on a keto diet long enough, your body gets into a state called ketosis. What is ketosis? Ketosis is a bit complicated to explain in full, but to be short and simple, **ketosis** is a process.

Ketogenesis sets in when the body has been low on carbohydrates for a time long enough to stave the brain of glucose. Since glucose is considerably high in carbohydrates and carbohydrate has been drastically reduced in a keto diet. Hey! You do not have to panic about this; it is not like your brains are going to starve to death. Hahaha! So, what does the brain do when glucose which is the main source of fuel? It taps into the body's reserve of ketones to get energy for itself and the body to function properly.

You see, ketones can be seen as compounds that can be used as a substitute for insulin, or blood sugar. We can simply say ketones are compounds that the body produces in the liver with fat when the insulin in the blood is really low. Although your body produces ketones in the liver all the time, the availability of carbohydrates, proteins, and fats plays a significant role in determining the rate at which ketones are being produced.

When the amount of proteins and carbohydrate intake increases in your diet, ketogenesis slows down, thereby knocking you off ketosis. But on the other hand, to start in the ketosis state, protein, and carbohydrates will have to be replaced with a significant about of fat that is just enough to maintain the body's functions still. It takes about three days of a strict keto diet to set an average weighed person into a state of ketosis.

Well, I know you might be figuring an easy way out, perhaps you have been knocked off ketosis a couple of times, and you want an easy way to get back. You figured that you could just take the ketone supplement. But the truth is, no, you should stay away from ketone supplements if you want to induce a healthy state of ketosis.

Ketone supplements will truly hype up the number of ketones in your body. But with no low-carbohydrate diet stimulus, no significant increase in the net amount of ketone production, no reduction in insulin production, and no increase in the fat oxidation, then ketosis cannot set in.

So, to wrap things up about what keto diet really means, you can see it as a diet that allows your body to generate no matter how little fuels called ketones which are used to keep the body functioning. It is important to note that keto dieting is completely safe, and healthy. But just in case of any allergies or health complications, you are advised to speak with a health care provider - doctor. Perhaps keto diet might just be what you need to get you even healthier that you figured.

The whole idea of keeping your brain starving and switching from the use of insulin by the body to ketones can be a bit daunting.

But I can still assure you again that the keto diet is safe and completely natural.

Imagine a person who is starving, maybe someone got stranded, or lost with no food. The person would actually survive because of the ability of the body to switch to ketogenesis. That is why humans can go for a couple of days without food and still survive.

Although the keto diet is not about starving yourself but changing what you eat. So, that is about what the keto diet is. In our next chapter we will be discussing the types of keto diet there is. Now that you know what a keto diet is, it is expedient that you are aware of the different types so that you can be properly educated about it.

Chapter 2: Types of Keto Diet

In our previous chapter, we talked about what the keto diet is. We also explained that when the body is on a strict keto diet long enough, ketogenesis sets in and the body is placed in a ketosis state. This simply means that the body would switch from its usual use of insulin in the body to ketones, which are produced in the liver. This switch is caused as a result of the low glucose in the blood as a result of the low carbohydrate intake in the keto diet.

In this chapter, we are going to be talking about the various types of the keto diet. Yes, of course, there are different types of the keto diet. Even though the keto diet is just simply about putting the body in a state of ketosis, there are different ways of acquiring it.

There are different reasons why people would even want to start the keto diet in the first place. But whatever your reasons may be, either for better health or just to lose weight, there are various types of keto diet you can exploit to achieve either one of your reasons or all of your reasons for starting a keto diet.

Although there are numerous health benefits of the keto diet, there is still some controversy as to who can do the keto diet and who should not. Clearly, with the whole process that the keto diet puts your body in, there are definitely some people whose body might not just be compatible with the keto diet.

In our previous chapter, we talked about consulting with a doctor before venturing into the keto diet. So, I will still insist that you visit a health care provider before starting the keto diet most especially for people with complications. This chapter will basically be focused on the various types of keto diet there is.

Types of Keto Diet

There are four major types of the keto diet. All other types that may exist are all derivatives of these four major types of the keto diet. The various types of keto diet are determined based on the composition of the main classes of food, which are the carbohydrates, proteins, and fats. The difference in proportion is what brings about the different types of keto diet we now know today. So, without further ado, let's get straight into it.

Standard Keto Diet (SKD)

The standard keto diet is types of keto diet where you plan most of your meals and snacks on mostly fat. The idea is to have fat as the largest proportion in the meal than any other class of food. A classic standard keto diet should look like this:

The proportion of the Macronutrient in SKD:

Fats - 75%

Proteins - 15-20%

Carbohydrates - 5-10%

The fats in an SKD should be able to provide most of the calories that the body needs to stay functioning normally. The SKD has shown to help a lot of times in reducing the body's fats and provide better control of the body's blood sugar level. There are other several health benefits, but that will be discussed later in the book.

Cyclic Keto Diet (CKD)

The cyclic keto diet is a type of keto diet that cycles anyone on it in and out of ketosis while they can still enjoy a balanced diet on an off day. A typical CKD should be in the proportion below:

The proportion of the Macronutrient in CKD

On keto diet days

Fats - 75%

Proteins - 15-20%

Carbohydrates - 5-10%

Off keto diet days

Fats - 25%

Proteins - 25%

Carbohydrates - 50%

The CKD simply involves days when you are on a strict keto diet, then days you go off and eat higher quality carbohydrates. There's no doubt that on off days in a CKD, you would be knocked off the ketosis days. This is the whole essence of this CKD. For a complete CKD cycle, it involves 5 days of a strict traditional keto diet, and two days of non-keto diet to make up on the cycle. Alternatively, you can call it a week because it takes 7 days.

Targeted Keto Diet (TKD)

The targeted keto diet is a bit different from the other keto diet in a way. The TKD is popularly used among people with a very active lifestyle and athletes as well. The TKD has to be in the following proportion:

The proportion of the Macronutrient in TKD

Fats - 65-70%

Proteins - 20%

Carbohydrates - 10-15%

The TKD is mainly for a targeted set of people with a more active lifestyle like workouts. These people may still want to enjoy the benefits of a keto diet. Mostly before and after vigorous activity, mainly workout, an extra of 20-30grams of carbohydrates are usually consumed. But this would not knock the person off ketosis state as the carbs are burnt away during a workout.

High-Protein Keto Diet (HPKD)

The high-protein keto diet, just like all the other keto diets, also sets the body in ketosis. The only difference is that people tend to find it easier to follow this modified keto diet than the rest. The proportion of the macronutrients in this diet are so similar to a regular balanced diet that people hardly feel any change. The HPKD has to be in the following proportion:

The proportion of the Macronutrient in HPKD

Fats - 60-65%

Proteins - 30%

Carbohydrates - 5-10%

According to the proportion above, the HPKD allows you to eat more protein and less fat than the usual, standard keto diet. Although it might not be as effective as the standard keto diet, the HPKD still produces a noticeable result.

Having said all this about the various types of the keto diets, it is up to you to choose which one of them is best for you. Based on what each of the types of keto diet entails, it is plain and simple that who wants to have the fastest and effective result would go for the SKD. And people who are not too consistent can choose from either of the rest, depending on their lifestyle and eating pattern.

Chapter 3: Food to Eat and Those to Avoid

Having discussed the different types of the keto diet, I am pretty sure that you might have wrapped your fingers around what you are likely allowed to eat and what you are not in a keto diet. Did you just think carbohydrates as one of them? Damn right, carbs are one of the foods that is a big-no for anyone on a keto diet.

But while carbohydrates might be the main food to avoid, clearly, it isn't the only food to avoid. This is especially true when you want to stay in that ketosis state you worked so hard to get into. So, to avoid bouncing in and out of ketosis state, which would strongly retard your progress in general, let us learn the different types of food to eat and where to draw the lines.

So, in this chapter, I am going to be giving you a quick food list of food that you can easily reference anytime. All the foods I will be suggesting are all Ketogenic related, so read them, get familiar with them and start enjoying your keto diet rather than struggling with what food is what.

Foods to Eat while on a Keto Diet

Going on a strict keto diet would set you in a ketosis state. The main idea on what you can eat when in a ketosis state so that you do not get knocked off ketosis depends on the about of glucose in the food. Basically, starchy foods should be avoided. But the following list of food can be eaten when on a keto diet without having to worry about being knocked of ketosis.

Meat

Meats are great source of protein and are required by the body to repair worn out tissues. Having just the right percentage of meat in your diet is a perfect way to keep your body functioning and as well on a state of ketosis. Meats like red meat, chicken, turkey, ham, steak, sausage and bacon can all be safely eaten.

Fatty Fish

Fishes are also wonderful for someone on a keto diet. Fish is rich in omega 3 fatty acids, which can be used by the brain. You can consider eating fatty fish like trout, salmon, mackerel, and tuna.

Eggs

Although eggs are mainly known to be rich in protein, they also contain carbohydrates. But the number of carbohydrates can be neglected when considering being knocked off ketosis. So, when going to eggs, you can get out the omega-3 whole eggs, or pastured eggs.

Butter and Cream

Butter and cream are very rich in fats. And fat should always be the main class of food that is in the diet of anyone on keto. Butter or cream is an excellent choice to make, but when going for either of them, search for grass-fed, if possible.

Cheese

Cheese is rich in fat and protein and also an excellent choice for someone on a keto diet. Having a couple of cheeses in your diet will help your body functioning and producing those ketones needed by the body. When going for cheese, go for unprocessed cheeses like cheddar, cream, blue, goat, or mozzarella cheese.

Nuts and Seeds

It depends on the nuts and seed you are choosing, but generally, nuts and seed are not bad to be eaten by someone on a keto diet. Nuts and seeds that are low on carbohydrates like Chia seeds, almonds, walnuts, pumpkin seeds, and flax seeds are ideal.

Healthy Oil

Consuming oil when on a keto diet is good, but not all oil is healthy. For an effective result at the end of the day, consider consuming oils like olive oil, avocado oil, and coconut oil.

Avocado

Just like avocado oil can be consumed by anybody on a keto diet, whole avocados can be consumed as well. So, you can consider having whole avocados and fresh guacamole in your diet.

Low Carbohydrate Vegetables

For some micronutrients that are needed by our body, consider having a vegetable, but only low carbohydrate vegetable. Many green vegetables, onions, peppers, tomatoes, and so on can be considered.

Condiments

Condiments can also be referred to as spices, don't get it twisted. You can have salt, pepper, herbs, and other healthy spices when on a keto diet. These are all much healthier than your usual condiments.

Food to Stay Away From

Just like there is food that can be freely eaten by someone on a keto diet, there are also foods that should be avoided. These foods are bad for ketosis and can knock you off your goal.

Sugary Foods

Most sugary foods are high in glucose and glucose will retard the production of ketones. Therefore, avoid sugary foods like fruit juice, soda, ice-cream, candies, and cakes and so on.

Grains or Starches

Some grains are a good source of starch, but starchy food is a no-no for ketosis. Avoid foods like rice, pasta, wheat, cereal, and the like.

Fruits

Although fruits are very healthy, when on a keto diet, avoid all fruits because of its fructose which is otherwise known as fruit sugar. And sugar can knock you off ketosis. But small fruits like berries and strawberries can be eaten.

Legumes and Beans

Beans and legumes like peas, lentils, chicken peas, and kidney beans and so on, should not be eaten when on a keto diet.

Tubers and Roots Vegetables

Tubers and root vegetables are starchy foods, and you should stay clear from them while on a keto diet. Tubers and root vegetables include the likes of potatoes, carrots, parsnips, sweet potatoes, and more.

Diet and Low-Fat Products

Most diet and low-fat products are often highly processed, and they usually contain a high composition of carbohydrates.

Some Sauce or Condiments

Even though some condiments can be consumed when on a keto diet with no side effect, some condiments like sugar or unhealthy fats should be avoided.

Alcohols

When it comes to alcoholic beverages, well, like it or not, they are high in carbohydrates and if you really want to get the benefits of the keto diet, steer clear of alcoholic beverages.

Chapter 4: Carbohydrates, Fats, Oils, Protein, Vegetables and Fruits, Nuts and Seeds

Obviously, in our last chapter all these where mentioned. Some of them fell into the group of foods that can be eaten when on a keto diet, while others fell in the group of diets that should be avoided when on a keto diet.

I figured you must have been wondering why this food or why that food has to be one. The truth is I felt that pain too myself when I first found out some foods are out of bounds. Carbohydrates, Fats and Oils, Proteins, Vegetables and Fruits, Nuts and Seeds are the main classes of food we find ourselves eating every day.

Even though these classes of food are the main kind of food we eat day in day out on the keto diet, the gameplay changes in a way. Perhaps what used to have been like 70% proportion in our diet might be reduced to 30%. This reduction might not be because you want to starve yourself, but to concentrate on a particular nutrient to get the desired effect.

In this chapter, we are going to be educating ourselves with the effects that Carbohydrates, Fats and Oils, Proteins, Vegetables and Fruits, Nuts and Seeds play in a keto diet.

Carbohydrates

When you think about carbohydrates in the keto diet, think enemy. Why? Because, when there are carbohydrates in the body, ketosis will not set in. So, in whatever type of keto dieting you choose to have, the proportion of carbohydrates in your food has to be low.

Carbohydrates in themselves are not bad. In fact, carbohydrates supply the body with the energy it needs to properly function. When carbohydrates are taken away, it leaves the body with no choice but to improvise and find other means to supply the body with energy. And fat seems to be the next resort.

Avoid as many carbohydrates as you can, and if you are not an extremist and you find yourself in a compromising position to eat carbohydrates, eat as little as you can. Low carbohydrate foods, on the other hand, can be consumed even when on a keto diet. So, if you must eat carbohydrates, ensure it is a low-carb food.

Fats and Oils

When on a keto diet, fats and oils should make up the major part of the food being consumed. There are different types of fat, but only a few of them are really involved in a keto diet. Some fats are healthy while others are not.

Saturated fats are safe and can be eaten when on a keto diet. Some examples of saturated fats include butter, coconut oil, and lard and so on.

Monounsaturated fats are also safe and can be eaten when on a keto diet. Some examples of monounsaturated fats include olive oil, macadamia nuts, avocado oil and so on.

Polyunsaturated fats occur naturally in animal proteins, fatty fish and the likes and are safe for consumption even when on a keto diet.

Trans fats, on the other hand, are bad for your health and you should avoid them as much as you can. They mostly include processed fats - hydrogenation. Therefore, avoid all hydrogenated fats like margarine, even though they have a good shelf life they can cause severe heart diseases.

Proteins

When it comes to protein, pertaining what to consume on a keto diet, virtually almost all proteins can be considered for consumption. Well, except the proteins that is harmful to our health. Even though proteins are great and can be consumed even when on a keto diet, quantity also matters, so you may want to be moderate on that.

When it comes to choosing an animal protein to consume when on a keto diet, choose a protein that is either grass-fed, or pasture raised. Also, choose animal proteins that are darker in color than the lighter ones. Why? Because the darker animal proteins are richer in fat than the lighter ones.

So, in other to avoid being knocked off ketosis by too much protein in your diet, always try to balance things off with fattier dishes as well as sauces too.

Vegetables and Fruits

Some examples of vegetable and fruits being consumed when on a keto diet includes, cabbage, spinach, green pepper balls, raspberries, blackberries, yellow onions, broccoli, and so on. Vegetables play an important part in the keto diet. Some vegetable and fruits are considerably high in carbohydrates and low in nutrients. Such vegetables and fruits need to be scrapped out of the list of vegetables and fruits to consider eating when on a keto diet.

On the other hand, when considering the type of vegetables and fruits to eat, go for vegetables and fruits that are low in carbohydrates, but high in nutrients. When the vegetables are dark in color or leafy, then you should consider it.

Also, fruits or vegetables that grow underground like carrots, onions, and potatoes should also be avoided. This is because many of them are high in carbohydrates. Therefore, they must be limited and monitored.

Nuts and Seeds

When on a keto diet, most of the commonly consumed nuts and seeds include pecans, hazelnuts, Brazil nuts, macadamia nuts, walnuts, nut butters, and so on. Nuts are generally better consumed when they are roasted. Why? Because roasting it will remove any anti-nutrient present in it.

I know we all love peanuts but try and avoid them as much as you can, because they are legumes. Although nuts have fat in them in some cases, there are cases where carbohydrate composition of the nut is high. Therefore, it is important always to take note of the composition of the nuts.

Nut flours can also be a great source of proteins and can build up the amount of protein in our diet, really fast. So, you might want to keep this on your checklist. Some **fatty nuts that are low in carbohydrates** include pecans, Brazil nuts, and macadamia nuts.

Some **fatty nuts but moderate in carbohydrates** include walnuts, almonds, pine nuts, peanuts, and hazelnuts. Some **fatty nuts but high in carbohydrates** include cashew nuts, pistachios, and so on.

Chapter 5: Quick Ketogenic Breakfast Recipes

So far so good, we have been making steady progress. In chapter 1 we talked about what keto diet really means. And in chapter 2 we talked about the different types of keto diet there is. Chapter 3 was all about the foods we can eat and those we should avoid when on a keto diet. Then we discussed all things Carbohydrates, Fats and Oils, Proteins, Vegetables and Fruits, Nuts and Seeds in chapter 4.

The essence of the first chapter through chapter 4 was to get everyone, beginners or not, acquainted with what keto diet is all about. It was to build a solid foundation of what you should know before proceeding to the main topic of this book. And that is keto diet recipes. You see, having discussed everything keto so far, we should put everything we have been blabbing about into action.

Now, in chapter 5, we will be discussing quick ketogenic breakfast recipe options. This chapter will set you on the right path of what to eat in the morning when on a keto diet. So, I will be highlighting some really cool recipes you can try out at home or anywhere. There is definitely something for everyone.

If you're a fan of paleo, dairy-free, or egg free, or you're a vegetarian, or even prefer whole30, there is the perfect recipe here for you. What is really intriguing about all these keto diet recipes you're about to check out is that they all have under 10g of net carbohydrates per serving.

Keto Diet with Bread, Bagels, and Donuts:

Collagen Keto Bread

You will believe in miracles after eating this collagen keto bread with zero carbs. The collagen keto bread is a perfect choice to eat for breakfast especially when you are on a keto diet. The fact that it doesn't even take much time to prepare just makes it even more perfect for breakfast.

To make things a little more interesting with the collagen keto bread, you can smother it with butter or a low-carbohydrate strawberry jam. You can even make a sandwich out of it, with items like avocados, eggs, and bacon.

Rosemary Vegetarian Keto Bagels

For an on-the-go breakfast, you can consider the Rosemary Vegetarian Keto Bagels. It's really easy to make and a perfect choice for a keto diet breakfast. The spongy texture of the bagels is from the almond flour, psyllium husk, and xanthan gum. It makes the bagels mouthwatering.

You can enjoy this Rosemary Vegetarian Keto Bagels without worrying about carbohydrate content, as it contains only about 4.5 net carbohydrates. So, choose Rosemary Vegetarian Keto Bagels for your breakfast before heading out for the day.

Keto Chocolate Vegetarian Cake Donuts

If you are a fan of chocolate, who says you can't have it for breakfast, even when on a keto diet? You can still enjoy your tender keto chocolate vegetarian cake doughnuts anytime, and it's even perfect for breakfast.

You can amp this keto breakfast recipe up with a cup of tea or coffee. The recipe contains just fairly above 2 net carbohydrates per donut. So, you can ease your mind as they are completely guilt-free. For even more tasty recipe, you can try using grass-fed butter with coffee, and full-fat coconut milk rather than creamy cream on the glaze.

Keto Diet with Pancakes, Waffles, and Crepes

Fluffy Pancakes with Almond Flour

If pancakes are your thing, you can still have pancakes, even when on a keto diet. For a perfect breakfast keto diet recipe, try the fluffy pancakes with almond flour. The almond flour is used to reduce the overall carbohydrate load.

With a hint of cinnamon and vanilla in the pancakes, you can make a healthy keto breakfast for the family. Basically, the overall carbohydrate load is usually about 4.5 net per serving. So, if pancakes are your thing, keep enjoying.

Crepes with Coconut Flour

Crepes are delicious and a perfect meal to have as breakfast. There are several ways of making crepes. However, making it with coconut flour makes it the perfect keto breakfast recipe. These thin and light crepes are perfect. They're just right for when you need a perfect base for some low-sugar berries.

To make things more interesting and more into the full strict keto diet, use coconut milk rather than almond milk. There is just barely over 1 net carbohydrate per crepe.

Buttery Waffles with Coconut Flour

Now, who doesn't love waffles? Crispy waffles can still be enjoyed when on a keto diet if you eat them right. The easiest way to get that fluffy, crunchy waffle and still be in check for the carbohydrate load is by using non-dairy milk, eggs, and coconut flour.

The overall recipe is about 4 net carbohydrates per waffle, so the carbohydrate level is still in check. And if you want to have a diary choice in the recipe, you can consider using grass-fed butter with full-fat coconut milk.

Keto Diet with Eggs and Meat

Eggs and Bacon Fat Bomb

Well, if you can't have decent food with a high concentration of carbohydrates, at least you can have a diet with more of protein. This keto breakfast recipe makes use of eggs mixture and bacon.

And with just about 0.2 grams of carbohydrates per each wrap of the fat bomb. The eggs and bacon fat bomb are just the perfect meal to have for breakfast as they are keto friendly. You can spice things up by using avocado as the oil base for the fat bomb.

Tacos with Guacamole and Bacon

Why not enjoy your tacos with guacamole and Bacon's and still be in line with the proportion of the classes of food required for a perfect keto diet?

All you need to make this perfect keto breakfast recipe a reality is a gently pastured boiled egg, guacamole and couple it all with crispy bacon. This delicious combination will leave you asking for more, and the overall carbohydrates load is about 4 net carbohydrates per Taco.

Chapter 6: Delicious Ketogenic Lunch Recipes

One thing you need to bear in mind is that lunch is the time when the largest quantity of food is being eaten. Unlike in our previous chapter, where we discussed the different breakfast recipes you can try, and most of them being light food that can easily digest.

The reason why mostly light foods are advised to be eaten in the morning is that the body is just waking up and still undergoing detoxication. At this point, it is not advisable to eat something too heavy so that the body will not be stressed out, and at the same time, it is important to eat something no matter how little.

So, after eating something very light for breakfast, and engaging yourself in your daily activities, it is only logical to expect hunger during lunch hours. There will definitely be cravings just to eat whatever you can lay your hands on. I'm pretty sure you can even eat your boss at that time. But despite the cravings, you have to still watch what you eat, because of your current state of ketosis.

There are a couple really cool recipes I am going to be laying out now. You should try out any one of the choices that you feel would do it just the right way for you. I will be dividing each of the recipes into groups, just like I did in for breakfast.

Ketogenic Lunch Recipes that saves you Money and Time

Frittata Turkey Sausage

So, you can enjoy your lunch with your same classic Frittata made out of turkey. When you think of this Frittata turkey sausage recipe for a keto diet, imagine it as an Italian omelet. Because this recipe makes use of the beaten eggs, meat, cheese, cream and vegetables.

The right quantity of the classes of food in this Frittata turkey sausage makes it just perfect for a keto lunch. They are also large enough to fill your stomach and satisfy your craving. The best part about the Frittata is that it is versatile and can be used in several ways like eaten immediately; you can freeze it and eat it at a later time and so on.

Low-Carbohydrate Keto Lasagna

Lasagna is great and is worth considering for a keto lunch diet. But for Lasagna to be a perfect keto lunch diet, you may have to replace its heavy carbohydrate noodles with thin slices of zucchini. This swap would make the lasagna healthier and more in line with what you can eat when you are on a keto diet.

Apart from its health benefits, this low-carbohydrate keto lasagna is tastier, softer, and has a cheesy texture. Zucchini in your lasagna is rich in potassium, has low calories, antioxidants, and is easily digestible. You can prepare this lasagna ahead of time, and you can take it to work or anywhere, and eat as lunch.

Cauliflower Bake

You can make casserole put of cauliflower and use it as an excellent lunch with no back effect when on a keto diet. Cauliflower casserole bake is great, and it is more like having loads of baked potato, packed with gooey cream cheese, bacon, cheddar, cauliflower, and butter.

The cauliflower bake is one meal you need to consider having every time because of how delicious they are, plus they are also healthy. The main secret to having mouth-watering cauliflower bake is the use of green onions. Then to spice the whole recipe up, you can add different protein - talking about meat or whatever you prefer. Each time you make the cauliflower bake change the protein to make it seem like a different meal entirely.

Ketogenic Lunch Recipes with Grass Fed Beef

Cheeseburgers Portobello Buns

Hell yes, you can still have your delicious cheeseburger Portobello buns even when are on a keto diet. All you got to do is just make it the right way, and you are on your way to enjoying your favorite meal for lunch at any time. Enough of skipping backyard BBQ just because you want to remain in ketosis.

This recipe is a perfect substitute for those hamburger buns. Now you can enjoy cheeseburgers seasoned with Portobello mushrooms. Taking a closer look into the Portobello mushrooms, it is one of two dietary fiber types - chitan and beta-glucans. These fibers provide enough bulk of food to fill your stomach and make you feel satisfied.

Beberé Enchilada with Stuffed Peppers

Who told you that you have to stop enchiladas just because you are on a keto diet? This recipe will require you to replace those tortillas with stuffed bell pepper and the use of beberé. Other ingredients used in this recipe includes the likes of ginger, garlic, chili pepper, fenugreek, rue, basil and cardamom, which is just to mention a few of the many ingredients used.

The process of preparation is quite simple too, and the bottom line is that they are an excellent choice for lunch. The enchilada just gives away this mouth-watering lunch and makes you feel like you haven't had enough even after the 5th rounds. Plus you can add or sub cauliflower to the recipe, instead of rice to reduce the carbohydrates load.

Ketogenic Lunch Recipe with Chicken

Roasted Chicken Stack

A roasted chicken stack is worthy of your lunch. They are delicious and will fill your belly with just enough to last you through the afternoon. Chicken is generally yummy and is quite ideal for a perfect keto diet. The level of carbohydrates in a roasted chicken stack is considerably low enough to not knock you off ketosis.

To enjoy this roasted chicken stack recipe, you can roast the chicken thigh and place it on a bed of cabbage as you can also add some toppings, like the prosciutto crisps. They might not be the fastest meal to prepare, to have five servings ready, it might take up to an hour. But, the good thing about the roasted chicken stack is that it can be made in advance for lunch.

Chapter 7: Simple Ketogenic Dinner Recipes

Dinner at last and dinner is also a time when you also need to watch what you eat. Just like you watch what you eat in the morning, so likewise, you will need to watch what you eat at dinner before going to bed. Lunch is the only time of the day when everyone is given license to eat as much as they can, although it doesn't include eating anyone besides you as well.

For dinner, especially for someone in a keto diet, there are certain types of food you should avoid, and those that you can freely eat. Being on a keto diet might make your choice of dinner seem a bit limited. However, there are loads of dinner recipes you can try on your own that would be just perfect for any home.

In this chapter of this book, I will be discussing some recipes you can try out. They will be just perfect for dinner especially when you are on a keto diet. Also, I will be splitting the recipes into groups. So, whatever it is that your taste falls into, you can still get your delicious tastes in a perfect keto dinner recipe.

Ketogenic Dinner Recipes with Beef

Keto Mexican Shredded Beef

This keto Mexican shredded beef is one meal you really need to consider for your next dinner. What really gets me intrigued about this recipe is the fact that it is super easy to prepare and would be ready in no time. Imagine getting back home from a stressful day at work, feeling tired, stressed, and hungry, the keto Mexican's shredded beef might just be your savior out of your current situation.

They are perfect for people on a keto diet, and they are also quite healthy. The keto Mexican's shredded beef, coated with warm spice, and simmer in a pot to prepare this low carbohydrate meal. With roasted vegetables, guacamole and lettuce wrap to make the dish look even more attractive.

Streak Fajita Roll Up

Make a nice streak fajita roll up for dinner and enjoy the fresh and flavorful dish anytime and anywhere. It is very easy to prepare and won't take forever to get ready. I'm probably less than 30 minutes, your streak fajita roll up is ready.

To prepare this great keto dinner recipe, no tortilla is required. Take your time to sauté the pepper and onions, then roll them up in a strip of beef as you sear it around. That is pretty much all there is to do about the streak fajita roll-up. You can serve it with salsa or guacamole. Fry the vegetables and meat in olive oil instead. To make the recipe even more irresistible, use grass-fed beef and high-quality spices.

Ketogenic Dinner Recipes with Seafood

Ketogenic Shrimp Scampi

Ketogenic Shrimp Scampi is yet another recipe you can take advantage of to have a nice keto dinner. For the time of preparation, the shrimp gets a bit of flavorful and light upgrade to improve its taste. Then it gets spiralized with your vegetable noodles. Then it is cooked with shrimp and lemony sauce.

The beautiful thing about this recipe is that it can perfectly impress anyone. So, to get the best out of this recipe, use chicken stock that has been pasteurized rather than wine, also add some wild-caught shrimp, and make sure you make use of grass-fed butter to make the recipe as a whole standout.

Baked Salmon with Garlic and Butter in Foil

For an extra seafood recipe, you could try the baked salmon with garlic and butter. This fresh and flavorful recipe is perfect for dinner when on a keto diet. You just simply need to flaky some of those wild-caught salmon in what is called a buttery garlic lemon sauce.

It is really easy to make and does not take the whole evening to make. You just simply need to heat the butter sauce just a bit, and then you can now use the sauce to brush over the salmon. Then put the salmon in a foil and heat for a while to make it tender. You should also try the grass-fed ghee as they can withstand the heat in an oven - use it rather than butter to make the recipe irresistible.

Ketogenic Dinner Recipes with Chicken

Zucchini Noodles with Butter Chicken

This is one recipe you may want to consider having as your dinner when on a keto diet that has no side effects to distorting your ketosis balance. All you need is just a butter sauce and a big chunk of chicken, and you are good to go all the way.

To have this mouth-watering recipe ready in no time, quickly spiralized the noodles, and then cook the chicken in spice and butter. Then simmer the zucchini noodles in the sauce, and you are good to go. You have your tasty, satisfying dinner hot and ready to eat.

Chapter 8: Health Friendly Ketogenic Snacks

So, you on a keto diet and you do feel hungry occasionally, but then you do not want just to eat whatever. Eating whatever you get just because of the craving to eat might just set you off course, and the balance would be distorted. Therefore, for a case just like this, you can have some health friendly ketogenic snacks.

Right! Some snacks are health friendly. But note that not all snacks are healthy. In fact, some snacks are junk food. So, ensure you know the difference before venturing into the world of snacks, so you don't get a junk snack confused with a health friendly snack.

Since there are a couple of health-friendly snacks to choose from, I will be listing out as many scholars I can in this chapter. Because this chapter has been dedicated exclusively just to health friendly Ketogenic snacks. So without further ado, let us jump right into the list.

Beef Jerky: so what is so special about this snack? Well, this is one snack you can be sure does not contain many ingredients and to top it all is low on carbohydrates. This, therefore, means that this snack is healthy, and you can have this snack anytime while on a keto diet. Basically, just to give you a tip watch out for snacks especially those that contain a high amount of sugar. Sugar can kick up the number of carbohydrates.

Nut Butters or Nut and Seeds: Nuts are great when it comes to having them as a snack. But you also need to remember that we talked about some nuts, which are not in a keto diet-wise not great. Nuts like cashew, peanuts and the rest are to be avoided, because their carbohydrate composition is high. You should also stay away from nuts that are rich in polyunsaturated oil. Nuts are low in carbohydrates and high in fat, some nuts are great for a keto diet while others are not.

Dark Sweetened Stevia Chocolate: Chocolate is also another types of snack you can have, and the dark sweetened stevia chocolate should be your choice. When you want to have chocolate as a snack, make sure it contains at least 80% cocoa. If the amount of cocoa present in the chocolate is less than this, then it is probably made of more sugar, and the carbohydrate load would be too high for someone on a keto diet.

Seaweed Snacks: Seaweed snacks should also be considered a snack especially when on a keto diet. The seaweed snacks are basically low in carbohydrates, but you have to make sure no extra ingredients are added because those extra ingredients can add a massive amount of carbohydrates to the snack. You should also make sure that it does not have some weird flavor or massive oil in them. With all these in check, you can enjoy your crunch of seaweed snacks anytime.

Avocados: Did anyone ever tell you that avocados can be used as an excellent choice of snack? Well, if you did not know, now you know. Avocados are French choice for a snack, they are whole and quite easy to eat - you do not need to cook or process it. All you will probably need is just a little pepper and salt, and you are good to go. And maybe you can add a little olive oil as well, just to spice up things.

Sardines: If you are a seafood person, then you can consider choosing sardines as a snack. Sardines do not only contain low carbohydrate, but they also supply your body with some really healthy fat. And be sure when I tell you sardines are highly recommended for you when on a keto diet.

Pepperoni Slices: Though pepperoni slices are highly processed they can be eaten as a snack even when on a keto diet. But you might also want to watch out for the quality of these you munch down in your belly. And if possible, try to get the ones that are hormones free and organic. Apart from these checkpoints, you can enjoy your high fat cheese anytime, and anywhere as a snack.

Iced Coffee: You can still enjoy the fresh taste of an energizing cup of coffee, even when on a keto diet. Well, this is obviously only for you are a coffee fan. When you want to drink coffee even when on a keto diet, ensure that you stay away from adding sugar to the coffee. You can add full-fat milk if you do not like your coffee black. MCT oil powders can also be used, and cream too.

Kale Chips: To spice up things a little bit, have kale chips anytime as a snack. When buying the kale chips get the ones that do not contain sugar. And if you want to have a little adventure and fun time in the kitchen you can make the kale chips yourself. All you need to make the kale chips are basically, coconut, lard, ghee, and oil.

Chapter 9: A Perfect 7 Days Keto Diet

And now, here comes the best part of this book. A seven days plan for a keto diet. Nothing hurts a keto diet more like not knowing what to eat for a complete week. How would you feel about having a perfect seven days keto diet plan? Great right! I thought as much. All you may just need to do is to alter the days you eat Wi-Fi food if you like to use this plan for more than seven days.

All the essential nutrients that your body needs to function have all been put into consideration when choosing this meal. Therefore, you can ease your mind about this diet and know that I got you covered. I know it might not be so easy to follow up this timetable, but if you can just put in a little effort into it, you would end up enjoying it. So, without further ado, let us jump right into it.

Day 1

On day 1 you can expect a total of about 1775 calories, net carbohydrates of 18.5g, a net protein of 87g, and a net fat of 148g.

Breakfast: For breakfast, you can have 2 creamy cheese pancakes, 2 pieces of cooked bacon, and you can top it with a cup of coffee with 2 tablespoons of heavy cream.

Snack: For a snack you can consider having 12 pieces of raw almond.

Lunch: Since lunchtime is when you eat the most, consider having 2 creamy cheese pancakes, 4 slices of low-sugar deli ham, 2 slices of cheddar deli cheese, and 1 tablespoon of mayonnaise.

Snack: You can have a string of cheese for a snack.

Dinner: For dinner, an excellent choice would be 2 enchilada green meatballs, ¾ cup of cauliflower cheesy chipotle.

Dessert: For dessert, a raspberry cheesecake bar would do just fine.

Day 2

On day 2 you can expect a total of 1410 calories, net carbohydrates of 19g, a net protein of 85g, and a net fat of 113g.

Breakfast: For an excellent breakfast choice, have 1 serving cheese and ham frittata, and you can spice it up with a cup of coffee with 2 tablespoons of heavy cream.

Snack: ½ of an avocado with a little bit of pepper and salt would do the snack magic for you.

Lunch: For lunch, you can have 4 enchilada green meatballs

Snack: You can snack up with 2 strings of cheese after lunch.

Dinner: For dinner, have 1 ¾ cups of sausage, squash soup, and kale. And bring the recipe to life with 1 cheddar muffin and jalapeno.

Dessert: 1 raspberry cheesecake bar would do just fine.

Day 3

You can expect to have a total of 1619 calories, net carbohydrates of 16.5g, a net protein of 66g, and a net fat of 133g.

Breakfast: For a perfect breakfast, choose 2 creamy cheese pancakes, 2 pieces of cooked bacon, and a cup of coffee with 2 tablespoons of heavy cream.

Snack: Snack up with ½ avocado with a little blend of pepper and salt.

Lunch: For lunch, consider having 1 serving cheese and ham frittata, 2 cups of romaine lettuces chopped, and 2 tablespoons of Italian dressing.

Snack: Enjoy 12 delicious almonds for your snack.

Dinner: Your perfect dinner should be a ¾ cup of cauliflower cheesy chipotle, and 2 enchilada green meatballs.

Dessert: For dessert, just have a raspberry cheesecake bar.

Day 4

On day 4 you can expect to have a total of 1279 calories, net carbohydrates of 19g. A net protein of 58g, and a net fat of 95g.

Breakfast: For your breakfast, consider 1 serving cheese and ham frittata, 2 pieces of cooked bacon, and a cup of coffee with 2 tablespoons of heavy cream.

Snack: Enjoy 12 delicious raw almonds as your snack.

Lunch: For lunch, 1 ¾ cup of sausage, squash soup and kale would do just fine.

Snack: You can consider having ½ avocado spiced with a little pepper and salt.

Dinner: For dinner, 1 servicing fried chicken, 2 cups of romaine lettuces chopped, and 2 tablespoons of Italian dressing would be just perfect.

Dessert: A raspberry cheese-cake bar would do the dessert magic.

Day 5

On day 5 you can expect to have a total of 1669 calories, net carbohydrates of 20g, a net protein of 81g, and a net fat of 130g.

Breakfast: A perfect breakfast choice would include 2 pieces of creamy cheese pancakes, 2 pieces of cooked bacon, and a cup of coffee with 2 tablespoons of heavy cream.

Snack: ½ avocado with a little spice of pepper and salt would do just fine for the snack.

Lunch: 1 serving fried chicken is perfect for lunch.

Snack: 1 serving cheese and ham frittata

Dinner: For dinner, consider having ¾ cup of cauliflower cheesy chipotle, and 2 enchilada green meatballs

Dessert: 1 raspberry cheese-cake bar would do just fine for dessert.

Day 6

On day 6 expect to have a total of 1447 calories, net carbohydrates of 18g, a net protein of 86g, and a net fat of 114g.

Breakfast: For breakfast choose 1 serving cheese and ham frittata, 2 pieces of cooked bacon, and a cup of coffee with 2 tablespoons of heavy cream.

Snack: Snack up with 12 delicious raw almonds.

Lunch: For lunch, have4 enchilada green meatballs.

Snack: Choose 2 strings of cheese for your afternoon snack.

Dinner: 1 ¾ cups of sausage, squash soup and kale, 2 cups of romaine lettuces chopped, and 2 tablespoons of Italian dressing is just perfect for dinner.

Dessert: Enjoy a raspberry cheese-cake bar for dessert.

Day 7

On day 7 expect to have a total of 1712 calories, net carbohydrates of 19.5g, a net protein of 92g, and a net fat of 138g.

Breakfast: For your breakfast, choose 2 creamy cheese pancakes, 2 pieces of cooked bacon, and a cup of coffee with 2 tablespoons of heavy cream.

Snack: A string of cheese would do just fine for a snack.

Lunch: For lunch have ¾ cup of cauliflower cheesy chipotle, and 2 enchilada green meatballs.

Snack: You can have 12 delicious raw almonds for a snack

Dinner: For dinner, you can have 1 serving Jerk BBQ rib, and ½ cup of broccoli slaw.

Dessert: and a raspberry cheese-cake bar.

Chapter 10: FAQs About the Keto Diets

Having talked about everything keto diet and some really cool recipes you can try. With even a perfect seven days plan for a keto diet, I am pretty sure some of you still have some questions to ask. You can leave some questions at the comment section below where you got this book from, I would be more than glad to see you get answers.

But to answer some of the most frequently asked questions about the keto diet, I will like to include that in this chapter. Don't get all bossed up and say the keto diet is not perfect; that's why all sorts of questions are arising. Definitely, questions are bound to arise, mostly due to a misunderstanding. So I am going to clear most of the doubts many have about the keto diet. So without further ado:

Does the keto diet have side effects? Yes, there are side effects. Even though the keto diet is perfectly safe, there are still some minor side effects that are bound to arise from time to time. The side effects are mostly referred to as the keto flu. The keto flu may include some side effects like increased hunger, poor mental function, poor energy, loss of sleep, nausea, a decrease in exercise, and digestive discomfort. This is just to mention some of the most common side effects. There may be other adverse side effects if the person is not very healthy.

Would I ever be able to eat carbohydrates again? Of course yes, you would be able to eat carbohydrates still. However, it is important that you do not eat too many carbohydrates especially during the early stage of the keto dieting. More like the first 2-3 month in which you start the keto diet, carbohydrates intake must be significantly low. But after this period, you can increase your carbohydrates intake just a little bit and periodically not all the time.

Can I build muscles when on a keto diet? To be completely honest with you, you can build muscles when on a keto diet, but it would be very difficult. The keto diet is not specifically meant for building muscles, rather it was designed to get rid of excess fat in your body. So, if you are interested in building muscle, I would suggest a more moderate carbohydrate and enough protein in your meal rather than the keto diet.

How much protein can I eat? This question has been answered in Chapter 2 of this book, when we talked about the different types of the keto diet. But to quickly answer this question, an average of 35% carbohydrates can be consumed by a person on a keto diet. This amount of protein would not put your state of ketosis on the line.

There are many speculations that the keto diet is dangerous is this true? No, the keto diet is not dangerous. In fact, the keto diet is a natural process that occurs in humans, many of times without us even realizing it. The reason why people think the keto diet is dangerous is that they confuse ketosis with ketoacidosis. Ketoacidosis occurs in the case of uncontrolled diabetes. But for ketosis, it occurs naturally.

I am on a keto diet and I experience diarrhea and digestion issues, what should I do? Diarrhea and digestion issues are common side effects that people on a keto diet do face at times. It is completely normal, and there is no need for you to panic. Yes, you will have to deal with the discomfort it brings to you. But do not worry; this side effect usually passes away after about 3 to 4 weeks. But if after this period it still persists, then I suggest you add more vegetables to your diet. Vegetables are rich in magnesium and magnesium helps against constipation.

How do I help against constant tiredness and fatigue when on a keto diet? There is every tendency that when you are on a keto diet, you would constantly feel tired and fatigued. When you frequently feel tired and fatigued all the time, it means that you have not gotten to a full ketosis state and your body is not efficiently utilizing its ketones and fat. A way around this would be to simply reduce your carbohydrates intake so that your body would be able to utilize the ketones and fat more efficiently. You can also try supplements like ketones or MCT oils to help with the tiredness.

Why does my Urine have a fruity smell? Well, do not allow this to alarm you. The fact your urine has a fruity smell means that the keto diet is really having the right effect on your body. So, it is a completely natural process for it to smell fruity. Moreover, the fruity smell is as a result of the excretes the body passes out during ketosis.

My breath smells too, what should I do? When you notice your breath has a smell as well, just simply drink plenty of water. And if drinking water does damp the smell, try chewing gum, but make sure the gum is sugar-free.

Printed in June 2019
by Rotomail Italia S.p.A., Vignate (MI) - Italy